Flight of Fear
Understanding Avian Influenza

© Copyright 2024 by Ayobami Akangbe- All rights reserved.

This document is geared towards providing exact and reliable information in regard to the topic and issue covered. The publication is sold with the idea that the publisher is not required to render accounting, officially permitted, or otherwise, qualified services. If advice is necessary, legal or professional, a practiced individual in the profession should be ordered.

- From a Declaration of Principles which was accepted and approved equally by a Committee of the American Bar Association and a Committee of Publishers and Associations.

In no way is it legal to reproduce, duplicate, or transmit any part of this document in either electronic means or in printed format. Recording of this publication is strictly prohibited and any storage of this document is not allowed unless with written permission from the publisher. All rights reserved.

The information provided herein is stated to be truthful and consistent, in that any liability, in terms of inattention or otherwise, by any usage or abuse of any policies, processes, or directions contained within is the solitary and utter responsibility of the recipient reader. Under no circumstances will any legal responsibility or blame be held against the publisher for any reparation, damages, or monetary loss due to the information herein, either directly or indirectly.

Respective authors own all copyrights not held by the publisher.

The information herein is offered for informational purposes solely and is universal as so. The presentation of the information is without contract or any type of guarantee assurance.

The trademarks that are used are without any consent, and the publication of the trademark is without permission or backing by the trademark owner. All trademarks and brands within this book are for clarifying purposes only and are the owned by the owners themselves, not affiliated with this document.

Table of Contents

Introduction 5
Chapter One 7
    Origins of Avian Influenza 7
    The Biology of Bird Flu 9
    Types and Strains 11
Chapter Two 14
    Human Health Impacts 14
    Economic and Agricultural Consequences 16
    One Health Approach 18
Chapter Three 21
    Pandemic Preparedness and Response 21
    Societal Impact and Ethical Considerations 23
    International Cooperation and Governance 25
Chapter Four 28
    Regional Perspectives 28
    Community Engagement and Risk Communication 30
    Innovations in Surveillance and Diagnostics 31
Chapter Five 34
    One Health in Action 34
    Emerging Threats and Future Challenges 36
    Towards a Resilient Future 37
Chapter Six 39
    Preparedness Planning and Response Frameworks 39
    Vaccine Development and Deployment 40
    Antiviral Therapies and Treatment Options 41
Chapter Seven 43

    Risk Communication in Crisis 43
    Ethical Decision-Making in a Crisis 44
    Building Community Resilience 45
    Learning from Crisis 47
Conclusion 49

Introduction

In the shadowed realms of our interconnected world, where whispers of danger ride upon the wind, there exists a silent threat that hovers ominously above us: avian influenza. Welcome to the journey through the "Flight of Fear: Understanding Avian Influenza."

Imagine, if you will, a tranquil morning in the heart of rural Asia, where the sun lazily caresses the fields, and the gentle hum of life fills the air. Yet, amidst this serene backdrop, a deadly drama unfolds. In a humble poultry farm, nestled within the embrace of verdant fields, a virus silently lurks, poised to unleash its fury upon unsuspecting hosts.

In the dim light of dawn, a farmer, his weathered hands etched with the toil of generations, begins his daily ritual. Little does he know that today, fate has woven a different tapestry. As he tends to his flock, a solitary cough breaks the stillness—a harbinger of the invisible menace that has taken root within his cherished birds. This is ground zero, the genesis of a tale that stretches across continents and through the annals of time.

But why should we, nestled snugly in our urban enclaves, concern ourselves with the plight of a humble farmer and his feathered charges? The answer lies in the very essence of our shared existence. Avian influenza is not merely a rural affliction—it is a global threat, a specter that haunts the corridors of power and the quiet alleys of the everyday.

In "Flight of Fear," we embark upon a quest to unravel the mysteries of avian influenza, to peer beyond the veil of ignorance and fear, and to confront the stark realities that lie beneath. Our journey is twofold: to understand the significance and potential dangers of this insidious disease, and to arm ourselves with knowledge—the most potent weapon in our arsenal.

Through the lens of personal narrative, we are beckoned into a world where the boundaries between man and nature blur, where the delicate balance of life hangs in the balance. We witness the struggles of those on the front lines—the farmers, the healthcare workers, the scientists—who battle tirelessly against an adversary that knows no mercy.

But fear not, for in the face of darkness, there is always light. The purpose of this book is clear: to illuminate the shadows, to empower the reader with the tools they need to navigate the treacherous waters of avian influenza. From the depths of history to the cutting edge of science, we journey together, armed with curiosity and resolve.

So, dear reader, buckle up and prepare for a voyage like no other. "Flight of Fear" beckons—a journey of discovery, of enlightenment, and ultimately, of hope. For in understanding the dangers that lurk above, we unlock the power to shape our destiny—to soar above the clouds and conquer the fear that binds us. Welcome aboard.

Chapter One

Origins of Avian Influenza

In exploring the ominous specter of avian influenza, we must embark on a journey through the annals of time, tracing the virus's origins and its enduring impact throughout history. This chapter delves into the historical context of avian influenza, unraveling the threads that bind its past to its present manifestations.

Our voyage begins in the ancient tapestry of human civilization, where whispers of avian influenza echo across millennia. Historical records dating back to ancient Egypt and Greece hint at the presence of avian diseases afflicting both humans and birds. While the precise identity of these ancient scourges remains shrouded in mystery, their echoes serve as harbingers of the threat that would later emerge.

Amidst the progression of civilizations and the succession of empires, avian influenza persisted in its covert expansion throughout the world.. From the bustling markets of medieval Europe to the remote villages of Asia, outbreaks of avian disease left devastation in their wake, decimating poultry flocks and occasionally claiming human lives. Yet, in the absence of modern scientific understanding, these outbreaks were often attributed to mysterious forces or divine wrath, their true nature obscured by the veil of ignorance.

The dawn of the modern era brought with it unprecedented advances in science and medicine, illuminating the shadows of the natural world and revealing the hidden truths of avian influenza. In the late 19th century, pioneering scientists first identified the influenza virus, laying the foundation for our understanding of this enigmatic pathogen. Yet, even as the mysteries of influenza began to unravel, the role of birds in its transmission remained a puzzle waiting to be solved.

It was not until the early 20th century that the pieces of the puzzle began to fall into place. In 1918, the world was plunged into the depths of a global pandemic—the Spanish flu—a cataclysmic event that claimed the lives of millions and forever altered the course of history. Though the specific origins of the Spanish flu are unknown, it is commonly considered to have originated in avian reservoirs, emphasizing birds' critical role in influenza transmission to humans.

With the dawn of the age of air travel, the stage was set for avian influenza to spread its wings and soar across continents. Bird migration patterns, shaped by the changing seasons and the rhythms of the natural world, provided the perfect conduit for the virus to traverse vast distances and infiltrate new territories. From the tundra of the Arctic to the tropical rainforests of the Amazon, no corner of the globe was immune to the reach of avian influenza.

As the 20th century drew to a close, the world bore witness to a series of alarming outbreaks of avian influenza in both humans and poultry. In 1997, the emergence of the H5N1 strain in Hong Kong sent shockwaves through the global health community, signaling the dawn of a new era of avian influenza. Subsequent outbreaks in Asia, Europe, and beyond served as grim reminders of the persistent threat posed by this elusive virus.

Yet, amidst the darkness, glimmers of hope began to emerge. The advent of molecular genetics and advanced surveillance techniques ushered in a new era of understanding, empowering scientists to unravel the intricate genetic code of avian influenza and trace its evolutionary trajectory. With each breakthrough, the veil of uncertainty surrounding avian influenza was lifted ever so slightly, illuminating the path forward in the fight against this formidable foe.

As we stand on the precipice of a new chapter in the saga of avian influenza, the lessons of history serve as our guiding light. From the ancient civilizations of antiquity to the modern laboratories of the 21st century, the story of avian influenza is a testament to the resilience of the human spirit and the boundless potential of scientific inquiry. Yet, the challenges that lie ahead are daunting, and the stakes could not be higher.

The Biology of Bird Flu

As we delve deeper into the enigmatic world of avian influenza, it becomes imperative to understand the essence of the culprit behind this silent menace—the influenza virus. In this chapter, we embark on a journey through Virology 101, unraveling the intricate structure and behavior of the virus that lies at the heart of avian influenza.

At its core, the influenza virus is a marvel of simplicity and complexity intertwined. The virus, which is comprised of a mere eight RNA segments enclosed in a lipid envelope, exhibits an exceptional capacity for mutation and adaptation, enabling it to elude the immune system and continue its unrelenting progression within the avian population.

Central to the influenza virus's ability to wreak havoc lies its surface proteins—hemagglutinin (HA) and neuraminidase (NA). By binding to receptors on the cell surface, HA facilitates the virus's entry into host cells, whereas NA assists in the discharge of newly formed viral particles from infected cells. It is the interplay between these two proteins that dictates the virus's ability to infect and spread within avian hosts.

But why are birds particularly susceptible to influenza? Unique avian physiologies and the intimate relationships between birds and their environment provide the solution. Unlike mammals, birds possess a specialized respiratory system characterized by a unidirectional airflow and air sacs, which create an ideal environment for the replication and spread of influenza viruses within the avian respiratory tract.

Moreover, avian species frequently form large colonies, which presents abundant prospects for the transmission of the virus via respiratory secretions and close proximity. Migration patterns further compound the problem, as birds traverse vast distances, carrying the virus with them and seeding new outbreaks in their wake.

Transmission dynamics play a pivotal role in the perpetuation of avian influenza within bird populations and its occasional spillover into humans. Transmission within the avian realm predominantly transpires via direct contact with infected birds or their secretions, in addition to exposure to contaminated environments including poultry farms and water sources.

However, the virus's ability to jump the species barrier and infect humans is a cause for concern. While direct transmission from birds to humans is relatively rare, it can occur under certain circumstances, particularly in settings where humans come into close contact with infected birds, such as live poultry markets or backyard farms.

After establishing itself within the human population, the virus has the potential to swiftly disseminate via respiratory droplets discharged during actions such as coughing or sneezing, in addition to via contact with contaminated surfaces. Severe cases of avian influenza in humans can cause pneumonia, respiratory failure, and even mortality, whereas the majority of cases cause mild symptoms similar to those of seasonal flu.

It is essential to comprehend the transmission dynamics in order to prevent and control avian influenza outbreaks in human and avian populations. By implementing surveillance, early detection, and prompt intervention strategies, it is possible to impede the progression of the virus and ensure the protection of animal and human health.

Types and Strains

Certain strains of avian influenza loom larger and more menacing than others. Among these, H5N1 stands out as a formidable adversary, striking fear into the hearts of scientists and the general populace alike. In this chapter, we turn our gaze towards this deadliest of strains, delving into its origins, characteristics, and the profound implications it holds for human health.

First identified in the late 1990s amidst an outbreak in poultry farms across Asia, H5N1 quickly established itself as a potent threat to both avian and human populations. Characterized by its high mortality rate in infected birds and sporadic but severe cases in humans, this strain sent shockwaves through the global health community, sparking fears of a potential pandemic on par with the Spanish flu of 1918.

What sets H5N1 apart from other strains of avian influenza is its ability to cause severe disease and death in both birds and humans. Although the majority of avian influenza strains are generally non-pathogenic to humans, H5N1 has the potential to cause damage to the lower respiratory tract, resulting in pneumonia, respiratory failure, and in severe instances, mortality. The virus's propensity for rapid mutation and its ability to reassort with other influenza viruses only serve to heighten concerns about its pandemic potential.

Yet, H5N1 is not the only strain of avian influenza to command our attention. In recent years, another significant threat has emerged in the form of H7N9. In contrast to H5N1, which predominantly impacts poultry, H7N9 has exhibited a concerning capacity to directly infect humans, resulting in severe morbidity and, in certain instances, mortality. The emergence of H7N9 has raised alarms within the global health community, prompting renewed efforts to monitor and control the spread of this insidious virus.

As we confront the specter of H5N1 and H7N9, it becomes increasingly clear that variability and evolution are fundamental aspects of the avian influenza landscape. Like all viruses, avian influenza viruses undergo constant genetic changes through mutation and reassortment, giving rise to new strains with varying degrees of virulence and transmissibility. Understanding the mechanisms driving this variability is essential to predicting and mitigating the impact of future outbreaks.

At the heart of avian influenza's evolution lies the concept of antigenic drift and shift. Antigenic drift is a phenomenon characterized by progressive modifications in the viral genome that result in the advent of novel strains exhibiting modified surface proteins. These changes can result in reduced effectiveness of existing vaccines and antiviral drugs, complicating efforts to control the spread of the virus. In contrast, antigenic shift transpires when two distinct strains of influenza viruses invade the identical host cell and swap genetic material, thereby generating new strains that possess the capacity to cause a pandemic.

The ongoing battle against avian influenza is a testament to the resilience of the human spirit and the power of scientific inquiry. By employing vigilant monitoring, implementing strong biosecurity protocols, and conducting ongoing investigations into the genetic mechanisms of the virus, it is possible to maintain a proactive stance against this perpetual menace.

Chapter Two

Human Health Impacts

As we navigate the labyrinthine landscape of avian influenza, it becomes imperative to shine a spotlight on the human toll exacted by this insidious virus. This section presents a comprehensive examination of the public health responses, potential complications, and clinical presentations associated with avian influenza in humans. It illuminates the significant ramifications that this virus can impose on both individuals and public health infrastructure.

First and foremost, it is essential to understand the clinical symptoms of avian influenza in humans. Unlike the seasonal flu, which typically presents with mild symptoms such as fever, cough, and body aches, avian influenza can manifest as severe respiratory illness with rapid onset. Common symptoms include high fever, cough, sore throat, muscle aches, and difficulty breathing. Patients may develop pneumonia, acute respiratory distress syndrome (ARDS), multi-organ failure, or even pass away in severe cases. Early recognition and prompt medical intervention are critical to improving outcomes for patients infected with avian influenza.

However, the story does not end with the onset of symptoms. For many patients, avian influenza can lead to a cascade of complications, each more dire than the last. Pneumonia, a prevalent complication of avian influenza, manifests as pulmonary inflammation and compromised gas exchange. If untreated, it can culminate in respiratory failure and fatality. Acute respiratory distress syndrome (ARDS), a potentially fatal condition characterized by substantial fluid accumulation and severe inflammation of the airways, may also ensue. In such cases, mechanical ventilation and intensive care are required to sustain respiration. Other complications may include secondary bacterial infections, sepsis, and organ failure, all of which contribute to the elevated mortality associated with avian influenza infections.

In the face of such daunting challenges, public health responses play a pivotal role in preventing and controlling outbreaks of avian influenza. Central to these efforts is surveillance, the systematic monitoring of avian and human populations for signs of the virus's presence. Early detection allows for swift intervention measures, such as culling infected poultry flocks, implementing quarantine measures, and administering antiviral medications to affected individuals. In order to prevent the spread of the virus, public health agencies disseminate vital information to the general public, including travel advisories, vaccination campaigns, and guidance on proper hygiene practices.

In addition to surveillance and containment measures, vaccination plays a central role in preventing human infections with avian influenza viruses. While no vaccine is currently available for widespread use against avian influenza, research is ongoing to develop vaccines that can confer immunity against specific strains of the virus. Public health agencies, meanwhile, amass antiviral medications such as zanamivir and oseltamivir, which can prevent the further spread of the virus and mitigate the intensity and length of symptoms in infected individuals.

Despite these efforts, the specter of avian influenza looms large, presenting a formidable challenge to public health systems worldwide.

As we confront this global threat, it is essential to remain vigilant, to invest in research and surveillance infrastructure, and to foster international collaboration and cooperation in the fight against avian influenza. Only through collective action and unwavering determination can we hope to stem the tide of this deadly virus and safeguard the health and well-being of future generations.

Economic and Agricultural Consequences

As we delve into the multifaceted repercussions of avian influenza, it is impossible to ignore the profound impact it has on the poultry industry. In this chapter, we turn our attention to the economic toll exacted by avian influenza outbreaks, the disruptions they cause to global trade and commerce, and the far-reaching implications for food security and nutrition worldwide.

The poultry industry stands as one of the hardest-hit sectors in the wake of avian influenza outbreaks. As the virus spreads through poultry flocks with alarming speed, farmers are forced to cull infected birds and implement stringent biosecurity measures to contain the spread of the disease. The depletion of poultry stocks and the subsequent decline in demand for poultry products due to concerns about contamination cause substantial financial detriment to producers and farmers, endangering their means of subsistence and the industry's stability.

However, the impact of avian influenza extends far beyond the confines of the poultry farm, reverberating throughout the global economy. Outbreaks of avian influenza can trigger disruptions to international trade and commerce, as countries implement trade restrictions and import bans on poultry products from affected regions. These disruptions can have cascading effects across supply chains, affecting not only poultry producers but also related industries such as feed manufacturers, transportation providers, and retailers.

The ramifications of avian influenza on global trade are particularly pronounced in regions heavily reliant on poultry exports for economic growth and development. Among the leading exporters of poultry in the world, Thailand, the United States, and Brazil could incur substantial declines in market share and export revenue should an avian influenza outbreak occur. These losses can have far-reaching implications for national economies, affecting employment, foreign exchange earnings, and overall economic stability.

In addition to its economic impact, avian influenza raises profound food security concerns, threatening the availability and affordability of poultry products for millions of people around the world. Poultry is an indispensable provider of protein and vital nutrients for billions of individuals, especially in low-income and middle-income nations where alternative protein sources may be scarce. Poultry production and trade disruptions have the potential to worsen food insecurity and malnutrition, particularly among susceptible demographics including children, expectant women, and the elderly.

Moreover, avian influenza outbreaks can disrupt food supply chains, leading to shortages and price volatility in local markets. As consumer confidence wanes and demand for poultry products declines, farmers may struggle to recoup their losses, exacerbating financial hardship and undermining efforts to ensure food security and nutrition for all. In some cases, consumers may turn to alternative protein sources, further straining already fragile food systems and exacerbating existing inequalities in access to nutritious food.

In the face of these challenges, it is essential to adopt a multifaceted approach to mitigate the impact of avian influenza on the poultry industry, global trade, and food security. This approach should encompass early detection and rapid response measures to contain outbreaks, investment in biosecurity infrastructure and surveillance systems to prevent future outbreaks, and support for affected farmers and communities to rebuild and recover from the economic impacts of the disease.

Furthermore, international cooperation and collaboration are critical to addressing the global dimensions of avian influenza and safeguarding the health and well-being of populations around the world. Through interdisciplinary collaboration, it is possible to enhance resilience, establish sustainable food systems, and guarantee universal access to nutritious and secure food, notwithstanding the unparalleled difficulties presented by avian influenza outbreaks.

One Health Approach

The interconnection of human, animal, and environmental health is a fundamental aspect of the complex web of life, which is encapsulated in the principles of One Health.. In this chapter, we unravel the interconnectedness of health and explore the relevance of the One Health approach to combating avian influenza. By means of cooperation, environmental stewardship, and collective effort, it is possible to pave the way towards a future that is both healthier and more resilient for all.

The premise of the One Health approach is that human, animal, and ecosystem health are fundamentally interdependent and interconnected.

. In the case of avian influenza, this interconnectedness is readily apparent. Birds serve as both hosts and vectors for the virus, capable of transmitting it to humans and other animals through close contact or environmental contamination. As such, efforts to prevent and control avian influenza must transcend traditional disciplinary boundaries, encompassing expertise from fields such as human and veterinary medicine, ecology, environmental science, and public health.

At the core of the One Health approach lies collaboration and cooperation among a wide range of stakeholders, each contributing their distinct expertise and perspectives to address the given issue.. Interdisciplinary teams of scientists, researchers, veterinarians, healthcare providers, policymakers, and community leaders work together to develop holistic strategies for preventing, detecting, and responding to avian influenza outbreaks. By pooling resources, sharing data, and coordinating efforts across sectors, these collaborative initiatives maximize the impact of interventions and improve outcomes for both human and animal populations.

Environmental factors are of paramount importance in the dynamics of avian influenza as they exert significant influence over its transmission patterns and subsequent dissemination. Habitat destruction, climate change, and biodiversity loss can disrupt ecosystems and alter the behavior of migratory birds, affecting their interactions with domestic poultry and increasing the risk of viral spillover. Environmental conservation efforts, such as habitat restoration, wetland preservation, and sustainable land use practices, can help mitigate these risks by preserving natural habitats and minimizing human-wildlife interactions.

Moreover, environmental surveillance programs can provide early warning signals of impending avian influenza outbreaks, allowing for timely intervention measures to be implemented. By monitoring wild bird populations, water quality, and environmental conditions, scientists can identify hotspots of viral activity and implement targeted interventions to reduce the risk of transmission to domestic poultry and humans. This proactive approach to surveillance and prevention is essential to preventing future outbreaks and safeguarding public health.

In addition to its role in preventing avian influenza outbreaks, environmental conservation also offers co-benefits for human and animal health. Sanitary ecosystem services, including but not limited to fertile soil, pure air, and clean water, are indispensable for the maintenance of life and the provision of livelihoods. By promoting biodiversity, protecting natural habitats, and mitigating the impacts of climate change, environmental conservation efforts can enhance resilience to infectious diseases, improve food security, and promote overall well-being for communities around the world.

As we navigate the complex and interconnected challenges of avian influenza, the principles of One Health offer a guiding light, illuminating a path towards a more sustainable and harmonious future. By embracing collaboration, cooperation, and environmental stewardship, we can harness the collective wisdom of diverse disciplines and forge a united front against this formidable adversary. Together, we can build a world where health knows no boundaries, and all living beings thrive in harmony with nature.

Chapter Three

Pandemic Preparedness and Response

As we stand at the crossroads of history, facing the daunting specter of avian influenza, we would do well to heed the lessons of the past. Across the annals of time, pandemics and outbreaks of infectious diseases have beset humanity, leaving an indelible imprint on the collective consciousness of all. Through a critical analysis of these historical occurrences and the application of the insights they provide, we can enhance our readiness to confront the forthcoming obstacles.

An imperative lesson derived from history pertains to the criticality of timely identification and effective intervention in order to contain epidemics of contagious diseases. Throughout history, from the Black Death in the 14th century to the Spanish flu in 1918, instances of delayed action and complacency in the face of emergent threats have repeatedly resulted in catastrophic outcomes. In the context of avian influenza, surveillance and monitoring systems play a pivotal role in detecting outbreaks early, allowing for swift intervention measures to be implemented before the virus has a chance to spread.

In recent years, significant strides have been made in the development of surveillance and monitoring systems for avian influenza. Advances in technology, such as real-time polymerase chain reaction (PCR) testing and geographic information systems (GIS), have revolutionized our ability to track the spread of the virus and identify hotspots of activity. By monitoring wild bird populations, poultry farms, and live bird markets, scientists can detect outbreaks early and implement targeted control measures to prevent further spread.

Another key lesson from history is the critical importance of vaccination in controlling infectious diseases. Throughout history, vaccines have played a central role in eradicating smallpox, eliminating polio, and reducing the burden of diseases such as measles, mumps, and rubella. In the case of avian influenza, efforts to develop effective vaccines have been ongoing for decades, with researchers racing to create vaccines that can confer immunity against specific strains of the virus.

Despite some advancements, the development of vaccines against avian influenza continues to face formidable obstacles. A significant challenge lies in the considerable genetic variability demonstrated by the virus, which may introduce complexities into the development and effectiveness of vaccines. Moreover, the emergence of novel strains, such as H5N1 and H7N9, presents a moving target for vaccine developers, requiring constant vigilance and adaptability to stay one step ahead of the virus.

Despite these challenges, ongoing research efforts hold promise for the development of effective vaccines against avian influenza. Novel vaccine platforms, such as recombinant DNA technology and viral vector vaccines, offer new avenues for vaccine development that may overcome some of the limitations of traditional approaches. Moreover, international collaborations and partnerships between governments, academia, and industry are accelerating progress towards the goal of developing vaccines that can provide broad protection against avian influenza viruses.

Societal Impact and Ethical Considerations

As we navigate the complex landscape of avian influenza, it becomes evident that the impact of the disease extends far beyond its biological manifestations. In this chapter, we delve into the social repercussions of avian influenza outbreaks and explore how human responses are shaped by fear, stigma, equity, access, and cultural perspectives.

Fear and stigma often accompany outbreaks of infectious diseases, and avian influenza is no exception. The specter of a deadly virus lurking in our midst can evoke feelings of anxiety, uncertainty, and dread, leading to heightened levels of fear within affected communities. Moreover, the stigma associated with avian influenza can further exacerbate social tensions and discrimination, particularly towards those perceived to be at higher risk of infection, such as poultry workers, farmers, and individuals living in affected regions.

Equity and access emerge as central ethical dilemmas in the context of avian influenza outbreaks, particularly concerning vaccine distribution and healthcare access. Inequities in access to healthcare services, vaccines, and essential resources can exacerbate existing disparities and deepen social divides, leaving vulnerable populations at greater risk of infection and death. Moreover, the prioritization of vaccine distribution raises ethical questions about who should have access to limited vaccine supplies and how allocation decisions should be made to ensure fairness and equity for all.

Cultural perspectives exert a substantial influence on human responses to avian influenza and shape perceptions of the disease.

Cultural beliefs, practices, and traditions can influence attitudes towards poultry farming, food consumption, and healthcare-seeking behavior, impacting the spread of the virus and the effectiveness of control measures. Moreover, cultural stigma and taboos surrounding illness and death can hinder efforts to detect and respond to avian influenza outbreaks, leading to underreporting and delays in seeking medical care.

In the face of these social repercussions, it is essential to recognize the interconnected nature of health and society and adopt a holistic approach to addressing the human dimensions of avian influenza outbreaks. This approach should prioritize community engagement, education, and empowerment, fostering trust and collaboration between affected communities, healthcare providers, policymakers, and public health agencies. We can minimize the social and economic impact on affected populations while developing more effective strategies for preventing and controlling avian influenza outbreaks through the localization of interventions and the participation of communities in decision-making processes.

Moreover, endeavors to tackle issues of access and equity must be founded upon the tenets of solidarity, fairness, and justice. Vaccines and healthcare services should be distributed based on need rather than ability to pay or social status, ensuring that the most vulnerable members of society receive the protection and care they deserve. Moreover, investments in healthcare infrastructure, education, and social support systems are essential for building resilient communities that can withstand the challenges posed by avian influenza and other infectious diseases.

International Cooperation and Governance

As we navigate the global landscape of avian influenza, it becomes evident that effective responses to this formidable threat require coordinated efforts at the international level. In this chapter, we explore the roles of global health organizations, multilateral agreements, and the complexities of global cooperation in addressing avian influenza outbreaks.

Global health organizations, such as the World Health Organization (WHO) and the Food and Agriculture Organization of the United Nations (FAO), play pivotal roles in coordinating responses to avian influenza outbreaks. The WHO serves as the leading authority on public health issues, providing guidance, technical expertise, and support to countries affected by avian influenza. Through its Global Influenza Programme and International Health Regulations, the WHO works to strengthen surveillance and monitoring systems, facilitate information sharing, and coordinate response efforts across borders.

Similarly, the FAO plays a crucial role in addressing avian influenza from an agricultural perspective, working to prevent the spread of the virus among domestic poultry populations and mitigate its impact on food security and livelihoods. Through its Emergency Prevention System for Transboundary Animal and Plant Pests and Diseases (EMPRES), the FAO supports countries in enhancing biosecurity measures, conducting risk assessments, and implementing control strategies to prevent and control avian influenza outbreaks.

Multilateral agreements and frameworks provide a framework for addressing cross-border health threats such as avian influenza. The International Health Regulations (IHR), adopted by the WHO in 2005, serve as a legally binding instrument for preventing, detecting, and responding to public health emergencies of international concern, including infectious disease outbreaks. By promoting collaboration, information sharing, and capacity-building among member states, the IHR strengthens global preparedness and response efforts, reducing the risk of pandemics and ensuring a coordinated international response to health emergencies.

However, global cooperation in the face of avian influenza outbreaks is not without its challenges. The highly transmissible nature of the virus, coupled with the interconnectedness of modern society, presents formidable obstacles to containment and control efforts. Political tensions, resource constraints, and competing priorities can hinder efforts to coordinate responses and mobilize resources effectively, leading to gaps in surveillance, communication, and response capacity.

Moreover, the emergence of novel strains of avian influenza, such as H5N1 and H7N9, poses new challenges for global health organizations and multilateral agreements. The potential for these highly pathogenic strains to induce severe illness and mortality in humans has sparked apprehension regarding the likelihood of a worldwide pandemic. Addressing these challenges requires sustained investment in research and development, enhanced surveillance and monitoring systems, and strengthened collaboration between governments, international organizations, and the private sector.

Despite these challenges, avian influenza outbreaks also present opportunities for innovation, collaboration, and solidarity.

Technological advancements, including rapid diagnostic tests and next-generation sequencing, have significantly transformed our capacity to promptly identify and monitor the progression of the virus, thereby facilitating more precise and efficient interventions. Moreover, the global response to avian influenza outbreaks has galvanized international cooperation and solidarity, fostering partnerships and alliances that transcend national boundaries and political differences.

Chapter Four

Regional Perspectives

As we traverse the global landscape of avian influenza, it becomes evident that the challenges and responses to the disease vary significantly across different regions of the world. In this chapter, we delve into the unique characteristics of avian influenza in Asia, Africa, the Americas, Europe, and Oceania, exploring regional approaches to control and prevention.

In Asia, where many outbreaks of avian influenza originate, the disease poses significant challenges due to the dense population of both humans and poultry, as well as the close proximity between wild birds and domestic poultry. Countries in Asia have implemented a range of control measures, including culling infected poultry flocks, enhancing biosecurity measures on farms, and conducting mass vaccination campaigns to reduce the spread of the virus. However, challenges remain, including limited resources, weak healthcare systems, and cultural practices that facilitate viral transmission.

In Africa, efforts to combat avian influenza are complicated by the continent's specific vulnerabilities, including limited healthcare infrastructure, widespread poverty, and high rates of poultry production in backyard and informal settings. African countries have made strides in enhancing surveillance and monitoring systems, strengthening laboratory capacity, and implementing biosecurity measures to prevent the spread of the virus. However, ongoing challenges, such as limited access to vaccines and antiviral medications, pose significant obstacles to effective control and prevention efforts.

In the Americas, Europe, and Oceania, regional approaches to avian influenza control and prevention vary depending on factors such as geographic location, agricultural practices, and regulatory frameworks. In the Americas, countries have implemented robust surveillance and monitoring systems, early detection and rapid response mechanisms, and strict biosecurity measures to prevent the introduction and spread of the virus. In Europe, efforts to control avian influenza are guided by the European Union's comprehensive regulatory framework, which includes measures such as compulsory vaccination, movement restrictions, and surveillance programs. In Oceania, countries have focused on strengthening biosecurity measures at borders, enhancing surveillance and monitoring systems, and promoting awareness and education among poultry farmers and the public.

Despite regional differences, one common thread unites efforts to combat avian influenza worldwide: the importance of collaboration, coordination, and information sharing among countries and regions. Regional and international partnerships play a crucial role in enhancing surveillance and monitoring capabilities, facilitating the exchange of best practices and lessons learned, and mobilizing resources to support control and prevention efforts. By working together, countries can strengthen their collective response to avian influenza and reduce the global burden of the disease.

The challenges and responses to avian influenza vary across different regions of the world, reflecting the diverse socio-economic, cultural, and environmental contexts in which the disease occurs. While regional approaches may differ, collaboration, coordination, and information sharing are essential for effectively controlling and preventing avian influenza outbreaks worldwide. By learning from each other's experiences and leveraging regional and international partnerships, countries can strengthen their capacity to respond to the challenges posed by avian influenza and safeguard the health and well-being of humans and animals alike.

Community Engagement and Risk Communication

In the intricate tapestry of combating avian influenza, the role of local communities emerges as a crucial thread woven into the fabric of effective response efforts. In this chapter, we delve into the importance of community involvement, effective risk communication strategies, and the building of trust in fostering cooperation and resilience in the face of avian influenza outbreaks.

Local communities play a pivotal role in detecting and responding to avian influenza outbreaks, serving as the first line of defense against the spread of the virus. Through vigilant surveillance, early detection, and reporting of sick or dead birds, community members can help identify potential hotspots of viral activity and facilitate rapid response measures to prevent further spread. Moreover, community-based organizations, such as farmers' associations, women's groups, and youth clubs, can serve as valuable channels for disseminating information, mobilizing resources, and implementing control measures at the grassroots level.

Effective risk communication is essential for engaging and empowering communities in the fight against avian influenza. By providing clear, timely, and accurate information about the risks posed by the virus, as well as recommended preventive measures and response actions, health authorities can help build awareness, reduce anxiety, and encourage compliance with control measures. Moreover, tailored communication strategies that take into account the cultural, linguistic, and socio-economic characteristics of the target audience are more likely to resonate with community members and elicit desired behaviors.

Building trust and transparency are critical components of effective risk communication and community engagement during avian influenza outbreaks. Trust is the foundation upon which cooperation, collaboration, and collective action are built, and transparency is essential for maintaining credibility and credibility in the eyes of the public. Health authorities must be open and honest in their communication with communities, acknowledging uncertainties, addressing concerns, and providing regular updates on the evolving situation. By fostering trust and transparency, health authorities can enhance community cooperation, mobilize support, and facilitate effective response efforts.

Moreover, building trust and transparency requires meaningful engagement with communities, involving them in decision-making processes, and soliciting their input and feedback on response efforts. Community members should be empowered to participate in the design, implementation, and evaluation of interventions, ensuring that their voices are heard and their needs are addressed. By fostering a sense of ownership and investment in response efforts, health authorities can strengthen community resilience and sustainability in the face of avian influenza outbreaks.

Innovations in Surveillance and Diagnostics

In the ever-evolving battle against avian influenza, technological advancements and data sharing initiatives have emerged as powerful tools in enhancing surveillance, detection, and response efforts. In this chapter, we delve into the role of technology and data sharing in combating avian influenza, exploring how advances in surveillance technology, rapid diagnostic tests, and early warning systems are revolutionizing our ability to anticipate, detect, and mitigate outbreaks.

Advances in technology and data analytics have transformed the landscape of avian influenza surveillance, enabling more timely and accurate detection of outbreaks and facilitating targeted response efforts. Remote sensing technologies, such as satellite imagery and unmanned aerial vehicles (UAVs), provide valuable insights into environmental factors that may influence the spread of the virus, such as bird migration patterns, habitat destruction, and climate change. Moreover, real-time data sharing platforms, such as the Global Initiative on Sharing Avian Influenza Data (GISAID) and the Global Early Warning System for Major Animal Diseases (GLEWS+), enable rapid exchange of information between countries and regions, enhancing global collaboration and coordination in response efforts.

Rapid diagnostic tests play a crucial role in the early detection and confirmation of avian influenza infections, enabling prompt initiation of control measures to prevent further spread of the virus. Traditional diagnostic methods, such as virus isolation and serological testing, can be time-consuming and labor-intensive, delaying diagnosis and response efforts. Rapid diagnostic tests, such as polymerase chain reaction (PCR) assays and antigen detection kits, offer a faster and more efficient alternative, providing results in a matter of hours rather than days. Moreover, advances in point-of-care testing technologies, such as handheld devices and smartphone applications, are making rapid diagnostic testing more accessible and affordable in resource-limited settings.

Early warning systems play a crucial role in anticipating and mitigating outbreaks of avian influenza, enabling proactive response measures to be implemented before the virus has a chance to spread. Predictive modeling techniques, such as mathematical modeling and machine learning algorithms, use historical data on avian influenza outbreaks, environmental conditions, and host populations to forecast the likelihood of future outbreaks and identify high-risk areas. Early warning systems, such as the Global Early Warning and Response System for Avian Influenza (GLEWS-AI), provide timely alerts and recommendations to policymakers, public health authorities, and other stakeholders, enabling them to take preemptive action to prevent or mitigate the impact of outbreaks.

Chapter Five

One Health in Action

In the dynamic realm of avian influenza control and prevention, the One Health approach stands as a beacon of hope, emphasizing the interconnectedness of human, animal, and environmental health in addressing complex health challenges. In this chapter, we explore the transformative potential of One Health through the lens of case studies, interdisciplinary research initiatives, and strategies for scaling up interventions.

Case studies offer valuable insights into successful examples of One Health approaches to avian influenza control and prevention, showcasing the tangible impact of collaborative efforts across sectors. In Thailand, for example, the establishment of the National Avian Influenza Control Program in 2004 brought together government agencies, veterinarians, public health officials, and poultry farmers to implement integrated surveillance, vaccination, and biosecurity measures. As a result, the country successfully contained outbreaks of H5N1 avian influenza and reduced the risk of transmission to humans.

Similarly, in Vietnam, the One Health approach has been instrumental in controlling the spread of avian influenza and mitigating its impact on human health. Through collaborative efforts between the Ministry of Agriculture and Rural Development, the Ministry of Health, and international partners, Vietnam has implemented targeted surveillance and vaccination campaigns, strengthened laboratory capacity, and enhanced public awareness and education about the risks of avian influenza. These efforts have helped to reduce the incidence of human cases and minimize the economic losses associated with outbreaks.

Interdisciplinary research initiatives play a crucial role in advancing our understanding of avian influenza and developing innovative solutions to control and prevention. Projects such as the EcoHealth Alliance's PREDICT program, which aims to identify emerging infectious diseases at the human-animal interface, and the International Livestock Research Institute's (ILRI) One Health Research, Education, and Outreach Center, which focuses on zoonotic diseases in sub-Saharan Africa, exemplify the collaborative spirit of One Health research. By integrating diverse perspectives and expertise from fields such as epidemiology, virology, ecology, and social science, these initiatives generate actionable insights and inform evidence-based interventions to reduce the risk of avian influenza transmission.

Scaling up One Health interventions requires strategic planning, resource mobilization, and stakeholder engagement to ensure sustainability and impact. Strategies for scaling up may include strengthening cross-sectoral collaboration and coordination, integrating One Health principles into national health policies and strategies, and mobilizing funding from diverse sources to support implementation efforts. Moreover, capacity-building initiatives, such as training programs for healthcare workers, veterinarians, and environmental scientists, are essential for building the necessary skills and expertise to implement One Health approaches effectively.

Emerging Threats and Future Challenges

In the realm of infectious diseases, avian influenza is not an isolated phenomenon but rather part of a broader landscape of zoonotic diseases with pandemic potential. In this chapter, we explore the zoonotic potential of other infectious diseases and their intersection with avian influenza. Additionally, we assess the impact of climate change and environmental factors on the spread and severity of avian influenza outbreaks, and discuss the threat of antimicrobial resistance in the context of avian influenza and its implications for treatment.

Other zoonotic diseases, such as Ebola virus disease, Middle East respiratory syndrome (MERS), and Zika virus, have demonstrated their capacity to cause widespread outbreaks with devastating consequences for human health, economies, and societies. Like avian influenza, these diseases originate in animals and can spill over into human populations through various pathways, including direct contact with infected animals, consumption of contaminated food products, and exposure to contaminated environments. By examining the zoonotic potential of other diseases, we gain valuable insights into the factors that contribute to spillover events and inform strategies for prevention, detection, and response.

Climate change and environmental factors play a significant role in shaping the dynamics of avian influenza outbreaks, influencing the distribution, abundance, and migratory patterns of avian species that serve as reservoirs for the virus. Changes in temperature, precipitation, and habitat availability can create favorable conditions for viral transmission and persistence, leading to increased risk of outbreaks in previously unaffected areas. Moreover, environmental degradation, deforestation, and urbanization can disrupt natural ecosystems and bring humans into closer contact with wildlife, increasing the likelihood of spillover events and emergence of novel strains of avian influenza.

Antimicrobial resistance poses a growing threat to the effectiveness of treatment and control measures for avian influenza, as well as other infectious diseases. The misuse and overuse of antimicrobial drugs in human and animal healthcare settings have led to the emergence of drug-resistant strains of avian influenza virus, compromising the efficacy of antiviral medications and vaccines. Moreover, the use of antimicrobial drugs in poultry production systems can select for resistant strains of avian influenza virus, further exacerbating the problem. Addressing antimicrobial resistance requires a multifaceted approach that includes stewardship of antimicrobial drugs, surveillance of resistance patterns, and development of alternative treatment strategies.

Towards a Resilient Future

In the ongoing battle against avian influenza and other pandemic threats, strengthening health systems is paramount. Investing in resilient health systems capable of responding swiftly and effectively to emerging health threats is essential to mitigate the impact of outbreaks. By bolstering surveillance, diagnostic capabilities, and response infrastructure, countries can detect and contain avian influenza outbreaks before they escalate into widespread pandemics. Moreover, building robust healthcare delivery systems, training healthcare workers, and ensuring access to essential medical supplies and resources are crucial for delivering timely care to those affected by avian influenza.

Research and development are critical for advancing our understanding of avian influenza and developing innovative solutions for prevention, treatment, and control. Areas for future research and innovation include the development of novel vaccines and antiviral medications, the identification of genetic markers associated with virulence and transmissibility, and the exploration of alternative control strategies such as gene editing and immune modulation. Moreover, interdisciplinary research initiatives that integrate human, animal, and environmental health perspectives can provide valuable insights into the complex dynamics of avian influenza transmission and inform evidence-based interventions to reduce the risk of outbreaks.

Collective responsibility is essential for addressing avian influenza and other pandemic threats effectively. Sustained global collaboration and solidarity are needed to coordinate response efforts, share information and resources, and mobilize support for affected countries. International organizations, such as the World Health Organization (WHO), the Food and Agriculture Organization of the United Nations (FAO), and the World Organisation for Animal Health (OIE), play a crucial role in facilitating collaboration and coordination among countries and regions. Moreover, partnerships between governments, non-governmental organizations, academia, and the private sector are essential for pooling expertise, resources, and innovation to address avian influenza and other global health challenges.

Chapter Six

Preparedness Planning and Response Frameworks

National preparedness plans are essential for guiding countries in their efforts to prevent, detect, and respond to avian influenza outbreaks. These plans outline strategies, policies, and procedures for surveillance, early detection, diagnosis, containment, and communication during outbreaks. They involve multiple stakeholders, including government agencies, public health authorities, veterinary services, and other relevant sectors, to ensure a coordinated and effective response. Preparedness plans are typically based on risk assessments, which identify potential threats and vulnerabilities, and prioritize actions to mitigate risks and enhance resilience.

Incident management systems are critical for coordinating response efforts during avian influenza outbreaks. These systems provide a structured framework for organizing, managing, and coordinating resources, personnel, and activities across multiple agencies and sectors. Incident management teams, comprising representatives from key stakeholders, such as health, agriculture, emergency management, and communications, work together to assess the situation, develop response plans, allocate resources, and communicate with the public. Incident management systems typically follow standardized protocols, such as the Incident Command System (ICS) or the Incident Management System (IMS), which facilitate interoperability and coordination among different entities.

Simulation exercises, such as tabletop exercises and simulations, play a vital role in testing and evaluating preparedness and response capabilities for avian influenza outbreaks. These exercises simulate real-life scenarios and allow stakeholders to practice response procedures, identify strengths and weaknesses, and refine plans and protocols. Tabletop exercises involve participants discussing and problem-solving through a hypothetical scenario, while simulations involve hands-on participation in a simulated environment. By conducting simulation exercises regularly, countries can enhance their readiness to respond to avian influenza outbreaks and improve coordination, communication, and decision-making among stakeholders.

Vaccine Development and Deployment

Vaccine production for avian influenza poses significant challenges due to the complex nature of the virus and the unique requirements of vaccine manufacturing and distribution. Avian influenza viruses are highly variable, with multiple subtypes and strains circulating in avian populations worldwide. Developing vaccines that provide broad protection against these diverse strains is challenging and requires extensive research, development, and testing. Moreover, vaccine production involves specialized facilities, equipment, and expertise, as well as stringent regulatory requirements to ensure safety, efficacy, and quality control. Scaling up production to meet global demand during outbreaks presents additional logistical and supply chain challenges, including vaccine formulation, packaging, storage, and distribution.

Numerous vaccine candidates for avian influenza are under development, ranging from traditional inactivated vaccines to newer technologies such as recombinant vaccines, virus-like particles, and DNA vaccines. These vaccine candidates target various components of the avian influenza virus, including the hemagglutinin (HA) and neuraminidase (NA) proteins, which play key roles in viral entry and replication. Promising vaccine candidates have shown efficacy in preclinical studies and early-phase clinical trials, demonstrating the potential to induce protective immune responses against avian influenza in humans and poultry. However, further research is needed to evaluate their safety, efficacy, and immunogenicity in larger clinical trials and real-world settings.

Optimal vaccination strategies for preventing avian influenza outbreaks depend on several factors, including the specific subtype and strain of the virus, the target population, and the epidemiological context. In poultry, vaccination strategies typically involve mass vaccination campaigns targeting domestic and commercial flocks to reduce the risk of viral transmission and minimize economic losses. These strategies may include routine vaccination, emergency vaccination in response to outbreaks, and strategic vaccination targeting high-risk areas or species. In humans, vaccination strategies focus on high-risk groups, such as poultry workers, healthcare workers, and individuals with underlying health conditions, to reduce the risk of zoonotic transmission and protect public health.

Antiviral Therapies and Treatment Options

Antiviral drugs play a crucial role in the treatment of avian influenza in humans, offering a means to reduce the severity and duration of symptoms, prevent complications, and improve clinical outcomes. Several antiviral drugs have been approved for the treatment of influenza, including neuraminidase inhibitors such as oseltamivir (Tamiflu) and zanamivir (Relenza), which work by blocking the activity of the influenza virus and inhibiting its replication. These drugs are most effective when initiated early in the course of illness, ideally within 48 hours of symptom onset, and are recommended for use in individuals with severe illness, underlying health conditions, or at high risk of complications from avian influenza.

In addition to approved antiviral drugs, several experimental therapies are being investigated for their potential to treat severe avian influenza infections and reduce mortality rates. These therapies include monoclonal antibodies, which target specific viral proteins and prevent viral entry into host cells, as well as immune modulators, which regulate the immune response and reduce inflammation and tissue damage. Other experimental approaches, such as RNA-based therapies, gene editing, and host-directed therapies, are also being explored for their ability to inhibit viral replication, enhance host immunity, and improve clinical outcomes in patients with severe avian influenza.

Despite the availability of antiviral drugs and experimental therapies, challenges remain related to access and equity in the treatment of avian influenza. Access to antiviral therapies may be limited in resource-constrained settings due to factors such as cost, availability, and infrastructure constraints. Moreover, during outbreaks, there may be increased demand for antiviral drugs, leading to shortages and inequities in access, particularly in low- and middle-income countries. Ensuring equitable distribution of antiviral therapies during outbreaks requires coordinated efforts among governments, international organizations, and pharmaceutical companies to prioritize allocation based on need, prioritize vulnerable populations, and promote transparency and accountability in decision-making processes.

Chapter Seven

Risk Communication in Crisis

Effective communication is essential during avian influenza outbreaks to inform the public, build trust, and mitigate the spread of misinformation and panic. Crisis communication principles provide a framework for communicating effectively during emergencies, emphasizing transparency, accuracy, empathy, and timeliness. Key principles include providing clear and consistent messaging, acknowledging uncertainties, addressing public concerns, and engaging with stakeholders to ensure that information is timely, relevant, and accessible. By adhering to these principles, public health authorities can enhance public understanding, cooperation, and compliance with preventive measures, ultimately reducing the impact of avian influenza outbreaks on human health and well-being.

Media engagement plays a critical role in disseminating accurate information and combating misinformation during avian influenza outbreaks. Journalists and media outlets play a key role in shaping public perceptions and behaviors, making them valuable partners in communication efforts. Strategies for engaging with the media include providing regular briefings and updates, responding promptly to media inquiries, and facilitating access to subject matter experts for interviews and commentary. Moreover, public health authorities should work collaboratively with the media to develop clear, concise, and engaging messaging that resonates with diverse audiences and encourages informed decision-making.

Addressing public concerns is essential for building trust and credibility during avian influenza outbreaks. Common concerns and fears may include fears of infection, mistrust of government authorities, skepticism about vaccine safety and efficacy, and concerns about the economic impact of control measures. Public health authorities should proactively address these concerns through targeted communication strategies, such as public service announcements, social media campaigns, and community outreach initiatives. By providing accurate information, addressing misconceptions, and empathizing with public concerns, public health authorities can foster trust, cooperation, and resilience in the face of avian influenza outbreaks.

Ethical Decision-Making in a Crisis

Ethical considerations surrounding resource allocation during avian influenza outbreaks are complex and challenging, requiring careful deliberation and decision-making to ensure fairness, equity, and transparency. Allocation of scarce resources, such as ventilators, personal protective equipment (PPE), and vaccines, involves balancing competing interests and priorities, including maximizing health outcomes, minimizing harm, promoting equity, and respecting individual rights and dignity. Ethical frameworks for resource allocation during outbreaks may include principles such as utilitarianism, which prioritizes the greatest good for the greatest number, and distributive justice, which emphasizes fairness and equitable distribution of resources based on need, vulnerability, and prognosis.

Triage protocols are essential for guiding clinical decision-making and resource allocation in healthcare settings during avian influenza outbreaks. These protocols prioritize patients based on severity of illness, likelihood of survival, and expected benefit from treatment, aiming to maximize the use of limited resources and save the most lives. Ethical frameworks for triage protocols may include principles such as medical necessity, which prioritizes patients with the greatest need for care, and proportionality, which considers the balance between potential benefits and harms of treatment. However, triage decisions can be ethically challenging, as they may involve difficult trade-offs between competing values, such as saving lives, respecting autonomy, and promoting justice.

Moral distress is a common experience among healthcare providers and other frontline workers during avian influenza outbreaks, resulting from the conflict between their professional duties and personal values in ethically challenging situations. Moral distress occurs when healthcare providers feel unable to act in accordance with their moral principles due to constraints, such as resource limitations, organizational policies, or systemic barriers. This can lead to feelings of guilt, frustration, and moral anguish, as healthcare providers grapple with difficult decisions, such as allocating scarce resources, providing care under challenging conditions, or prioritizing certain patients over others. Addressing moral distress requires organizational support, ethical guidance, and opportunities for reflection and debriefing to help healthcare providers cope with the emotional toll of ethical decision-making and maintain resilience in the face of adversity.

Building Community Resilience

Community-based approaches are crucial for building resilience to avian influenza outbreaks, empowering local communities to take ownership of their health and well-being. These approaches involve engaging with community members, leaders, and organizations to develop and implement tailored interventions that address local needs, priorities, and resources. Community-based initiatives may include education and awareness campaigns, training programs, capacity-building activities, and community mobilization efforts to promote preventive measures, early detection, and effective response to avian influenza outbreaks. By fostering collaboration, participation, and empowerment, community-based approaches can enhance community resilience, reduce vulnerability, and strengthen social cohesion in the face of outbreaks.

Social support networks play a vital role in helping communities cope with the impacts of avian influenza outbreaks, providing emotional, practical, and informational support to individuals and families affected by the disease. These networks may include family members, friends, neighbors, religious groups, community organizations, and health and social service providers who offer assistance, solidarity, and companionship during times of crisis. Social support networks can help mitigate the psychosocial impacts of avian influenza outbreaks, such as anxiety, fear, and social isolation, by providing a sense of belonging, connection, and reassurance. By fostering social support networks, communities can promote resilience, coping, and recovery in the aftermath of outbreaks.

Psychological first aid is a critical component of psychosocial support for individuals and communities affected by avian influenza outbreaks, providing immediate and practical assistance to address their emotional and psychological needs. Psychological first aid involves providing compassionate, non-judgmental support, listening actively, validating emotions, and offering practical assistance to help individuals cope with stress, grief, trauma, and other psychological challenges. It emphasizes safety, comfort, and empowerment, respecting individual autonomy, culture, and preferences. Psychological first aid may be provided by trained professionals, such as mental health professionals, social workers, and community volunteers, who offer support in a variety of settings, including healthcare facilities, shelters, and community centers. By offering psychological first aid, communities can promote resilience, recovery, and healing in the aftermath of avian influenza outbreaks.

Community-based approaches, social support networks, and psychological first aid are essential components of psychosocial support for individuals and communities affected by avian influenza outbreaks. By fostering collaboration, participation, and empowerment, community-based approaches can enhance community resilience and reduce vulnerability to outbreaks. Social support networks play a vital role in providing emotional, practical, and informational support to individuals and families affected by the disease, promoting resilience and coping. Psychological first aid offers immediate and compassionate assistance to address the emotional and psychological needs of individuals and communities affected by avian influenza outbreaks, promoting recovery and healing. Through these interventions, communities can strengthen their capacity to cope with the psychosocial impacts of outbreaks and emerge stronger and more resilient in the face of adversity.

Learning from Crisis

Post-outbreak evaluation is crucial for assessing the effectiveness of response efforts and identifying lessons learned to inform future preparedness and response efforts. These evaluations involve reviewing the response activities, identifying strengths and weaknesses, and making recommendations for improvement. By conducting thorough evaluations, public health authorities and policymakers can identify gaps in preparedness, response capacity, and coordination, as well as areas for improvement in surveillance, communication, and resource allocation. Post-outbreak evaluations also provide an opportunity to engage stakeholders, gather feedback, and build consensus on priorities for strengthening health systems and improving pandemic preparedness.

Adaptation and innovation are essential for responding to evolving threats and challenges posed by avian influenza outbreaks. Lessons learned from past outbreaks can inform future preparedness and response efforts, guiding the development of innovative strategies, technologies, and interventions to enhance resilience and mitigate the impact of future outbreaks. By fostering a culture of continuous learning, adaptation, and innovation, public health authorities, researchers, and policymakers can anticipate emerging risks, identify novel solutions, and build adaptive capacity to respond effectively to evolving threats. This may include investing in research and development, leveraging new technologies, and engaging with diverse stakeholders to foster collaboration and innovation in pandemic preparedness and response.

Resilience building is a multifaceted process that involves strengthening individual, community, and societal capacity to withstand and recover from adverse events, including avian influenza outbreaks. Strategies for building resilience may include enhancing access to healthcare services, promoting preventive measures, such as vaccination and hand hygiene, fostering social cohesion and community networks, and addressing underlying social determinants of health, such as poverty, inequality, and environmental degradation. By investing in resilience-building efforts, public health authorities and policymakers can reduce vulnerability, enhance adaptive capacity, and promote sustainable development, ultimately improving the health and well-being of individuals and communities.

Conclusion

As we come to the conclusion of our journey through the complex landscape of avian influenza, it is essential to reflect on the key takeaways and insights gleaned from our exploration. Throughout this book, we have delved into the origins, transmission dynamics, clinical manifestations, and public health responses to avian influenza, gaining a deeper understanding of this persistent global threat. We have examined the interconnectedness of health systems, the importance of community involvement, and the ethical considerations surrounding resource allocation and triage protocols during outbreaks. Moreover, we have explored the role of technology, data sharing, and innovation in enhancing surveillance efforts and early detection of avian influenza outbreaks.

Looking ahead, the future of avian influenza research and prevention holds both challenges and opportunities. Continued investment in research, surveillance, and vaccine development is essential to stay ahead of evolving strains and mitigate the risk of future pandemics. Additionally, strengthening health systems, enhancing global collaboration, and promoting One Health approaches are critical for addressing the complex interplay of factors driving the emergence and spread of avian influenza.

As we reflect on the global impact of avian influenza, it is clear that our collective response to this challenge requires concerted action and collaboration across borders, sectors, and disciplines. By advocating for policies and practices that promote global health security, we can help build a more resilient world capable of withstanding and recovering from infectious disease threats.

Despite the daunting challenges posed by avian influenza and other infectious diseases, we remain optimistic about humanity's ability to overcome adversity and build a brighter future. Through ongoing collaboration, innovation, and preparedness, we can mitigate the impact of avian influenza and other global health threats, safeguarding the health and well-being of current and future generations.

In closing, I urge each of you to take an active role in building a more resilient and prepared world for the challenges that lie ahead. Whether through advocacy, research, or community engagement, each of us has a role to play in shaping the future of global health. Together, we can work towards a world where the threat of avian influenza and other infectious diseases is minimized, and where health and well-being are prioritized for all.

www.ingramcontent.com/pod-product-compliance
Lightning Source LLC
Chambersburg PA
CBHW070420230526
45471CB00006B/2902